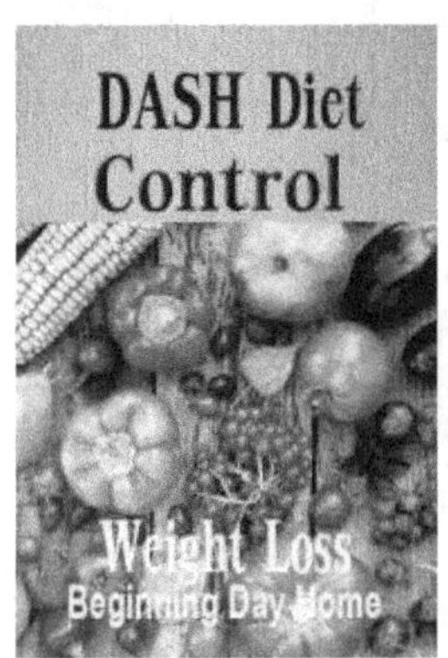

DASH Diet Control

Beginning Day Home Weight Loss Programme Possible Control Pressure Live Healthy Heart Disease Ensuring Clean

Diseases. We need to control eating.,The pattern control is very

Eating Easy To Recipesn Cooking Planning Beginning Of You Life & Family

You will begin to see results within a few weeks to months.

1 Week DASH Diet Base Control .... Calories

Date	Breakfast	Lunch	Dinner	Snacks	DASH Diet
					Base On.............Calories
MONDAY					Note.......................
TUESDAY					Fruits................. Vegetables............
					Fat free Lowfat Milk dairy............
WEDNESDAY					Whole Grains ....
THURSDAY					Lean Meat Fish &Poultry...............
					Nut Seeds & Legumes.............
FRIDAY					Oils...................... ....
					Sweets Salt.......... Alcohol...............
SATURDAY					
					Gaols Success Base Planer Calories..................
SUNDAY					

1 Week DASH Diet Base Control .... Calories				

Date	Breakfast	Lunch	Dinner	Snacks	DASH Diet Base On.............Calories
MONDAY					Note........................
TUESDAY					
WEDNESDAY					
THURSDAY					
FRIDAY					
SATURDAY					
SUNDAY					

1 Week DASH Diet Base Control .... Calories					
Date	Breakfast	Lunch	Dinner	Snacks	DASH Diet Base On............Calories Note......................
MONDAY					
TUESDAY					
WEDNESDAY					
THURSDAY					
FRIDAY					
SATURDAY					
SUNDAY					

Date	Breakfast	Lunch	Dinner	Snacks	DASH Diet Base On.............Calories Note.........................
MONDAY					
TUESDAY					
WEDNESDAY					
THURSDAY					
FRIDAY					
SATURDAY					
SUNDAY					

Date	Breakfast	Lunch	Dinner	Snacks	DASH Diet Base On..........Calories Note......................
MONDAY					
TUESDAY					
WEDNESDAY					
THURSDAY					
FRIDAY					
SATURDAY					
SUNDAY					

1 Week DASH Diet Base Control .... Calories

1 Week DASH Diet Base Control .... Calories					
Date	Breakfast	Lunch	Dinner	Snacks	DASH Diet Base On.............Calories
MONDAY					Note........................
TUESDAY					
WEDNESDAY					
THURSDAY					
FRIDAY					
SATURDAY					
SUNDAY					

1 Week DASH Diet Base Control .... Calories

Date	Breakfast	Lunch	Dinner	Snacks	DASH Diet Base On............Calories
MONDAY					Note.........................
TUESDAY					
WEDNESDAY					
THURSDAY					
FRIDAY					
SATURDAY					
SUNDAY					

1 Week DASH Diet Base Control .... Calories

Date	Breakfast	Lunch	Dinner	Snacks	DASH Diet Base On.............Calories
MONDAY					Note........................
TUESDAY					
WEDNESDAY					
THURSDAY					
FRIDAY					
SATURDAY					
SUNDAY					

<table>
<tr><td colspan="6">1 Week DASH Diet Base Control.. Calories</td></tr>
<tr><td>Date</td><td>Breakfast</td><td>Lunch</td><td>Dinner</td><td>Snacks</td><td>DASH Diet
Base On...........Calories</td></tr>
<tr><td>MONDAY</td><td></td><td></td><td></td><td></td><td>Note......................</td></tr>
<tr><td>TUESDAY</td><td></td><td></td><td></td><td></td><td></td></tr>
<tr><td>WEDNESDAY</td><td></td><td></td><td></td><td></td><td></td></tr>
<tr><td>THURSDAY</td><td></td><td></td><td></td><td></td><td></td></tr>
<tr><td>FRIDAY</td><td></td><td></td><td></td><td></td><td></td></tr>
<tr><td>SATURDAY</td><td></td><td></td><td></td><td></td><td></td></tr>
<tr><td>SUNDAY</td><td></td><td></td><td></td><td></td><td></td></tr>
</table>

1 Week DASH Diet Base Control .... Calories					

Date	Breakfast	Lunch	Dinner	Snacks	DASH Diet Base On.............Calories
MONDAY					Note........................
TUESDAY					
WEDNESDAY					
THURSDAY					
FRIDAY					
SATURDAY					
SUNDAY					

1 Week DASH Diet Base Control .... Calories					
Date	Breakfast	Lunch	Dinner	Snacks	DASH Diet Base On............Calories
MONDAY					Note.........................
TUESDAY					
WEDNESDAY					
THURSDAY					
FRIDAY					
SATURDAY					
SUNDAY					

1 Week DASH Diet Base Control .... Calories

Date	Breakfast	Lunch	Dinner	Snacks	DASH Diet Base On..........Calories
MONDAY					Note........................
TUESDAY					
WEDNESDAY					
THURSDAY					
FRIDAY					
SATURDAY					
SUNDAY					

1 Week DASH Diet Base Control .... Calories

Date	Breakfast	Lunch	Dinner	Snacks	DASH Diet Base On............Calories
MONDAY					Note.........................
TUESDAY					
WEDNESDAY					
THURSDAY					
FRIDAY					
SATURDAY					
SUNDAY					

1 Week DASH Diet Base Control .... Calories					
Date	Breakfast	Lunch	Dinner	Snacks	DASH Diet Base On............Calories
MONDAY					Note........................
TUESDAY					
WEDNESDAY					
THURSDAY					
FRIDAY					
SATURDAY					
SUNDAY					

1 Week DASH Diet Base Control .... Calories

Date	Breakfast	Lunch	Dinner	Snacks	DASH Diet Base On............Calories
MONDAY					Note......................
TUESDAY					
WEDNESDAY					
THURSDAY					
FRIDAY					
SATURDAY					
SUNDAY					

1 Week DASH Diet Base Control .... Calories				

Date	Breakfast	Lunch	Dinner	Snacks	DASH Diet Base On............Calories
MONDAY					Note........................
TUESDAY					
WEDNESDAY					
THURSDAY					
FRIDAY					
SATURDAY					
SUNDAY					

1 Week DASH Diet Base Control .... Calories					
Date	Breakfast	Lunch	Dinner	Snacks	DASH Diet Base On............Calories
MONDAY					Note........................
TUESDAY					
WEDNESDAY					
THURSDAY					
FRIDAY					
SATURDAY					
SUNDAY					

1 Week DASH Diet Base Control .... Calories

Date	Breakfast	Lunch	Dinner	Snacks	DASH Diet Base On............Calories
MONDAY					Note........................
TUESDAY					
WEDNESDAY					
THURSDAY					
FRIDAY					
SATURDAY					
SUNDAY					

1 Week DASH Diet Base Control				.... Calories	

Date	Breakfast	Lunch	Dinner	Snacks	DASH Diet Base On............Calories
MONDAY					Note........................ ....
TUESDAY					
WEDNESDAY					
THURSDAY					
FRIDAY					
SATURDAY					
SUNDAY					

1 Week DASH Diet Base Control .... Calories

Date	Breakfast	Lunch	Dinner	Snacks	DASH Diet
					Base On............Calories
MONDAY					Note........................
TUESDAY					
WEDNESDAY					
THURSDAY					
FRIDAY					
SATURDAY					
SUNDAY					

1 Week DASH Diet Base Control					.... Calories

Date	Breakfast	Lunch	Dinner	Snacks	DASH Diet Base On............Calories
MONDAY					Note......................
TUESDAY					
WEDNESDAY					
THURSDAY					
FRIDAY					
SATURDAY					
SUNDAY					

1 Week DASH Diet Base Control .... Calories					
Date	Breakfast	Lunch	Dinner	Snacks	DASH Diet Base On............Calories
MONDAY					Note........................
TUESDAY					
WEDNESDAY					
THURSDAY					
FRIDAY					
SATURDAY					
SUNDAY					

1 Week DASH Diet Base Control .... Calories

Date	Breakfast	Lunch	Dinner	Snacks	DASH Diet Base On............Calories
MONDAY					Note......................
TUESDAY					
WEDNESDAY					
THURSDAY					
FRIDAY					
SATURDAY					
SUNDAY					

1 Week DASH Diet Base Control .... Calories

Date	Breakfast	Lunch	Dinner	Snacks	DASH Diet
					Base On............Calories
MONDAY					Note.........................
TUESDAY					
WEDNESDAY					
THURSDAY					
FRIDAY					
SATURDAY					
SUNDAY					

Date	Breakfast	Lunch	Dinner	Snacks	DASH Diet

1 Week DASH Diet Base Control .... Calories

DASH Diet
Base On..........Calories

Note.......................

MONDAY

TUESDAY

WEDNESDAY

THURSDAY

FRIDAY

SATURDAY

SUNDAY

1 Week DASH Diet Base Control				.... Calories	
Date	Breakfast	Lunch	Dinner	Snacks	DASH Diet Base On............Calories
MONDAY					Note........................
TUESDAY					
WEDNESDAY					
THURSDAY					
FRIDAY					
SATURDAY					
SUNDAY					

| 1 Week DASH Diet Base Control | | | | | .... Calories |

Date	Breakfast	Lunch	Dinner	Snacks	DASH Diet Base On............Calories
MONDAY					Note......................
TUESDAY					
WEDNESDAY					
THURSDAY					
FRIDAY					
SATURDAY					
SUNDAY					

Date	Breakfast	Lunch	Dinner	Snacks	DASH Diet Base On.............Calories
MONDAY					Note........................
TUESDAY					
WEDNESDAY					
THURSDAY					
FRIDAY					
SATURDAY					
SUNDAY					

1 Week DASH Diet Base Control .... Calories

1 Week DASH Diet Base Control .... Calories					
Date	Breakfast	Lunch	Dinner	Snacks	DASH Diet Base On.............Calories
MONDAY					Note........................
TUESDAY					
WEDNESDAY					
THURSDAY					
FRIDAY					
SATURDAY					
SUNDAY					

| 1 Week DASH Diet Base Control | | | | .... Calories |
| | | | | |

Date	Breakfast	Lunch	Dinner	Snacks	DASH Diet Base On............Calories
MONDAY					Note........................ ....
TUESDAY					
WEDNESDAY					
THURSDAY					
FRIDAY					
SATURDAY					
SUNDAY					

1 Week DASH Diet Base Control .... Calories					
Date	Breakfast	Lunch	Dinner	Snacks	DASH Diet Base On.............Calories
MONDAY					Note.........................
TUESDAY					
WEDNESDAY					
THURSDAY					
FRIDAY					
SATURDAY					
SUNDAY					

1 Week DASH Diet Base Control .... Calories					
Date	Breakfast	Lunch	Dinner	Snacks	DASH Diet Base On.............Calories
MONDAY					Note......................
TUESDAY					
WEDNESDAY					
THURSDAY					
FRIDAY					
SATURDAY					
SUNDAY					

1 Week DASH Diet Base Control .... Calories

Date	Breakfast	Lunch	Dinner	Snacks	DASH Diet Base On............Calories
MONDAY					Note........................ ....
TUESDAY					
WEDNESDAY					
THURSDAY					
FRIDAY					
SATURDAY					
SUNDAY					

1 Week DASH Diet Base Control .... Calories

Date	Breakfast	Lunch	Dinner	Snacks	DASH Diet
					Base On.............Calories
MONDAY					Note.........................
TUESDAY					
WEDNESDAY					
THURSDAY					
FRIDAY					
SATURDAY					
SUNDAY					

1 Week DASH Diet Base Control .... Calories					
Date	Breakfast	Lunch	Dinner	Snacks	DASH Diet Base On.............Calories
MONDAY					Note........................
TUESDAY					
WEDNESDAY					
THURSDAY					
FRIDAY					
SATURDAY					
SUNDAY					

1 Week DASH Diet Base Control .... Calories

Date	Breakfast	Lunch	Dinner	Snacks	DASH Diet Base On............Calories
MONDAY					Note........................
TUESDAY					
WEDNESDAY					
THURSDAY					
FRIDAY					
SATURDAY					
SUNDAY					

1 Week DASH Diet Base Control					.... Calories
Date	Breakfast	Lunch	Dinner	Snacks	DASH Diet Base On............Calories Note........................
MONDAY					
TUESDAY					
WEDNESDAY					
THURSDAY					
FRIDAY					
SATURDAY					
SUNDAY					

1 Week DASH Diet Base Control .... Calories

Date	Breakfast	Lunch	Dinner	Snacks	DASH Diet Base On............Calories
MONDAY					Note......................
TUESDAY					
WEDNESDAY					
THURSDAY					
FRIDAY					
SATURDAY					
SUNDAY					

1 Week DASH Diet Base Control .... Calories					
Date	Breakfast	Lunch	Dinner	Snacks	DASH Diet Base On............Calories
MONDAY					Note........................
TUESDAY					
WEDNESDAY					
THURSDAY					
FRIDAY					
SATURDAY					
SUNDAY					

1 Week DASH Diet Base Control .... Calories					
Date	Breakfast	Lunch	Dinner	Snacks	DASH Diet Base On............Calories
MONDAY					Note........................
TUESDAY					
WEDNESDAY					
THURSDAY					
FRIDAY					
SATURDAY					
SUNDAY					

1 Week DASH Diet Base Control .... Calories

Date	Breakfast	Lunch	Dinner	Snacks	DASH Diet Base On.............Calories
MONDAY					Note......................
TUESDAY					
WEDNESDAY					
THURSDAY					
FRIDAY					
SATURDAY					
SUNDAY					

1 Week DASH Diet Base Control .... Calories					

Date	Breakfast	Lunch	Dinner	Snacks	DASH Diet Base On............Calories
MONDAY					Note......................... ....
TUESDAY					
WEDNESDAY					
THURSDAY					
FRIDAY					
SATURDAY					
SUNDAY					

1 Week DASH Diet Base Control .... Calories					

Date	Breakfast	Lunch	Dinner	Snacks	DASH Diet Base On............Calories
MONDAY					Note.........................
TUESDAY					
WEDNESDAY					
THURSDAY					
FRIDAY					
SATURDAY					
SUNDAY					

1 Week DASH Diet Base Control .... Calories

Date	Breakfast	Lunch	Dinner	Snacks	DASH Diet
					Base On............Calories
MONDAY					Note.........................
TUESDAY					
WEDNESDAY					
THURSDAY					
FRIDAY					
SATURDAY					
SUNDAY					

1 Week DASH Diet Base Control .... Calories

Date	Breakfast	Lunch	Dinner	Snacks	DASH Diet Base On............Calories
MONDAY					Note.........................
TUESDAY					
WEDNESDAY					
THURSDAY					
FRIDAY					
SATURDAY					
SUNDAY					

1 Week DASH Diet Base Control .... Calories					
Date	Breakfast	Lunch	Dinner	Snacks	DASH Diet Base On.............Calories
MONDAY					Note.........................
TUESDAY					
WEDNESDAY					
THURSDAY					
FRIDAY					
SATURDAY					
SUNDAY					

1 Week DASH Diet Base Control .... Calories

Date	Breakfast	Lunch	Dinner	Snacks	DASH Diet Base On............Calories
MONDAY					Note........................
TUESDAY					
WEDNESDAY					
THURSDAY					
FRIDAY					
SATURDAY					
SUNDAY					

1 Week DASH Diet Base Control .... Calories

Date	Breakfast	Lunch	Dinner	Snacks	DASH Diet Base On............Calories
MONDAY					Note......................... ....
TUESDAY					
WEDNESDAY					
THURSDAY					
FRIDAY					
SATURDAY					
SUNDAY					

1 Week DASH Diet Base Control .... Calories

Date	Breakfast	Lunch	Dinner	Snacks	DASH Diet
					Base On.............Calories
					Note........................
MONDAY					
TUESDAY					
WEDNESDAY					
THURSDAY					
FRIDAY					
SATURDAY					
SUNDAY					

Date	Breakfast	Lunch	Dinner	Snacks	DASH Diet
MONDAY					Base On............Calories Note........................
TUESDAY					
WEDNESDAY					
THURSDAY					
FRIDAY					
SATURDAY					
SUNDAY					

1 Week DASH Diet Base Control .... Calories

1 Week DASH Diet Base Control.. Calories					
Date	Breakfast	Lunch	Dinner	Snacks	DASH Diet Base On............Calories Note...................... ....
MONDAY					
TUESDAY					
WEDNESDAY					
THURSDAY					
FRIDAY					
SATURDAY					
SUNDAY					

1 Week DASH Diet Base Control				.... Calories	
Date	Breakfast	Lunch	Dinner	Snacks	DASH Diet Base On.............Calories
MONDAY					Note..........................
TUESDAY					
WEDNESDAY					
THURSDAY					
FRIDAY					
SATURDAY					
SUNDAY					

1 Week DASH Diet Base Control .... Calories

Date	Breakfast	Lunch	Dinner	Snacks	DASH Diet Base On............Calories
MONDAY					Note......................
TUESDAY					
WEDNESDAY					
THURSDAY					
FRIDAY					
SATURDAY					
SUNDAY					

1 Week DASH Diet Base Control.. Calories					

Date	Breakfast	Lunch	Dinner	Snacks	DASH Diet Base On............Calories
MONDAY					Note......................... ....
TUESDAY					
WEDNESDAY					
THURSDAY					
FRIDAY					
SATURDAY					
SUNDAY					

1 Week DASH Diet Base Control .... Calories

Date	Breakfast	Lunch	Dinner	Snacks	DASH Diet Base On............Calories Note........................
MONDAY					
TUESDAY					
WEDNESDAY					
THURSDAY					
FRIDAY					
SATURDAY					
SUNDAY					

1 Week DASH Diet Base Control .... Calories

Date	Breakfast	Lunch	Dinner	Snacks	DASH Diet Base On............Calories
MONDAY					Note........................
TUESDAY					
WEDNESDAY					
THURSDAY					
FRIDAY					
SATURDAY					
SUNDAY					

1 Week DASH Diet Base Control .... Calories					

Date	Breakfast	Lunch	Dinner	Snacks	DASH Diet Base On.............Calories
MONDAY					Note........................
TUESDAY					
WEDNESDAY					
THURSDAY					
FRIDAY					
SATURDAY					
SUNDAY					

1 Week DASH Diet Base Control				.... Calories	
Date	Breakfast	Lunch	Dinner	Snacks	DASH Diet Base On............Calories
MONDAY					Note.........................
TUESDAY					
WEDNESDAY					
THURSDAY					
FRIDAY					
SATURDAY					
SUNDAY					

1 Week DASH Diet Base Control .... Calories					
Date	Breakfast	Lunch	Dinner	Snacks	DASH Diet Base On...........Calories
MONDAY					Note........................ ....
TUESDAY					
WEDNESDAY					
THURSDAY					
FRIDAY					
SATURDAY					
SUNDAY					

1 Week DASH Diet Base Control .... Calories					

Date	Breakfast	Lunch	Dinner	Snacks	DASH Diet Base On............Calories
MONDAY					Note.........................
TUESDAY					
WEDNESDAY					
THURSDAY					
FRIDAY					
SATURDAY					
SUNDAY					

1 Week DASH Diet Base Control .... Calories					
Date	Breakfast	Lunch	Dinner	Snacks	DASH Diet Base On............Calories Note........................
MONDAY					
TUESDAY					
WEDNESDAY					
THURSDAY					
FRIDAY					
SATURDAY					
SUNDAY					

1 Week DASH Diet Base Control				.... Calories	
Date	Breakfast	Lunch	Dinner	Snacks	DASH Diet Base On.............Calories
MONDAY					Note........................
TUESDAY					
WEDNESDAY					
THURSDAY					
FRIDAY					
SATURDAY					
SUNDAY					

1 Week DASH Diet Base Control .... Calories					
Date	Breakfast	Lunch	Dinner	Snacks	DASH Diet Base On...........Calories
MONDAY					Note........................ ....
TUESDAY					
WEDNESDAY					
THURSDAY					
FRIDAY					
SATURDAY					
SUNDAY					

1 Week DASH Diet Base Control .... Calories					

Date	Breakfast	Lunch	Dinner	Snacks	DASH Diet Base On............Calories
MONDAY					Note........................
TUESDAY					
WEDNESDAY					
THURSDAY					
FRIDAY					
SATURDAY					
SUNDAY					

1 Week DASH Diet Base Control					.... Calories
Date	Breakfast	Lunch	Dinner	Snacks	DASH Diet Base On.............Calories
MONDAY					Note........................
TUESDAY					
WEDNESDAY					
THURSDAY					
FRIDAY					
SATURDAY					
SUNDAY					

1 Week DASH Diet Base Control .... Calories					
Date	Breakfast	Lunch	Dinner	Snacks	DASH Diet Base On............Calories
MONDAY					Note........................
TUESDAY					
WEDNESDAY					
THURSDAY					
FRIDAY					
SATURDAY					
SUNDAY					

1 Week DASH Diet Base Control... Calories					
Date	Breakfast	Lunch	Dinner	Snacks	**DASH Diet** Base On............Calories
MONDAY					Note........................
TUESDAY					
WEDNESDAY					
THURSDAY					
FRIDAY					
SATURDAY					
SUNDAY					

| 1 Week DASH Diet Base Control | | | | .... Calories |

Date	Breakfast	Lunch	Dinner	Snacks	DASH Diet Base On..........Calories
MONDAY					Note......................
TUESDAY					
WEDNESDAY					
THURSDAY					
FRIDAY					
SATURDAY					
SUNDAY					

1 Week DASH Diet Base Control .... Calories					

Date	Breakfast	Lunch	Dinner	Snacks	DASH Diet Base On.............Calories
MONDAY					Note........................
TUESDAY					
WEDNESDAY					
THURSDAY					
FRIDAY					
SATURDAY					
SUNDAY					

1 Week DASH Diet Base Control .... Calories

Date	Breakfast	Lunch	Dinner	Snacks	DASH Diet Base On............Calories
MONDAY					Note........................
TUESDAY					
WEDNESDAY					
THURSDAY					
FRIDAY					
SATURDAY					
SUNDAY					

1 Week DASH Diet Base Control					.... Calories
Date	Breakfast	Lunch	Dinner	Snacks	DASH Diet Base On............Calories
MONDAY					Note........................ ....
TUESDAY					
WEDNESDAY					
THURSDAY					
FRIDAY					
SATURDAY					
SUNDAY					

1 Week DASH Diet Base Control .... Calories

Date	Breakfast	Lunch	Dinner	Snacks	DASH Diet Base On.............Calories
MONDAY					Note.........................
TUESDAY					
WEDNESDAY					
THURSDAY					
FRIDAY					
SATURDAY					
SUNDAY					

1 Week DASH Diet Base Control				.... Calories	

Date	Breakfast	Lunch	Dinner	Snacks	DASH Diet
MONDAY					Base On............Calories Note........................
TUESDAY					
WEDNESDAY					
THURSDAY					
FRIDAY					
SATURDAY					
SUNDAY					

1 Week DASH Diet Base Control .... Calories					
Date	Breakfast	Lunch	Dinner	Snacks	DASH Diet Base On............Calories Note........................
MONDAY					
TUESDAY					
WEDNESDAY					
THURSDAY					
FRIDAY					
SATURDAY					
SUNDAY					

1 Week DASH Diet Base Control .... Calories

Date	Breakfast	Lunch	Dinner	Snacks	DASH Diet Base On............Calories
MONDAY					Note......................
TUESDAY					
WEDNESDAY					
THURSDAY					
FRIDAY					
SATURDAY					
SUNDAY					

1 Week DASH Diet Base Control					.... Calories
Date	Breakfast	Lunch	Dinner	Snacks	DASH Diet Base On............Calories
MONDAY					Note.........................
TUESDAY					
WEDNESDAY					
THURSDAY					
FRIDAY					
SATURDAY					
SUNDAY					

1 Week DASH Diet Base Control .... Calories					
Date	Breakfast	Lunch	Dinner	Snacks	**DASH Diet** Base On............Calories
MONDAY					Note........................
TUESDAY					
WEDNESDAY					
THURSDAY					
FRIDAY					
SATURDAY					
SUNDAY					

1 Week DASH Diet Base Control .... Calories

Date	Breakfast	Lunch	Dinner	Snacks	DASH Diet Base On............Calories
					Note.........................
MONDAY					
TUESDAY					
WEDNESDAY					
THURSDAY					
FRIDAY					
SATURDAY					
SUNDAY					

1 Week DASH Diet Base Control .... Calories					

Date	Breakfast	Lunch	Dinner	Snacks	DASH Diet Base On...........Calories
MONDAY					Note........................
TUESDAY					
WEDNESDAY					
THURSDAY					
FRIDAY					
SATURDAY					
SUNDAY					

1 Week DASH Diet Base Control .... Calories

Date	Breakfast	Lunch	Dinner	Snacks	DASH Diet Base On............Calories
MONDAY					Note............................
TUESDAY					
WEDNESDAY					
THURSDAY					
FRIDAY					
SATURDAY					
SUNDAY					

1 Week DASH Diet Base Control .... Calories					
Date	Breakfast	Lunch	Dinner	Snacks	DASH Diet Base On............Calories
MONDAY					Note.........................
TUESDAY					
WEDNESDAY					
THURSDAY					
FRIDAY					
SATURDAY					
SUNDAY					

1 Week DASH Diet Base Control .... Calories					
Date	Breakfast	Lunch	Dinner	Snacks	**DASH Diet** Base On.............Calories Note.........................
MONDAY					
TUESDAY					
WEDNESDAY					
THURSDAY					
FRIDAY					
SATURDAY					
SUNDAY					

1 Week DASH Diet Base Control .... Calories					
Date	Breakfast	Lunch	Dinner	Snacks	DASH Diet Base On............Calories
MONDAY					Note...................... ....
TUESDAY					
WEDNESDAY					
THURSDAY					
FRIDAY					
SATURDAY					
SUNDAY					

1 Week DASH Diet Base Control.. Calories					
Date	Breakfast	Lunch	Dinner	Snacks	**DASH Diet** Base On.............Calories Note........................
MONDAY					
TUESDAY					
WEDNESDAY					
THURSDAY					
FRIDAY					
SATURDAY					
SUNDAY					

1 Week DASH Diet Base Control .... Calories

Date	Breakfast	Lunch	Dinner	Snacks	DASH Diet Base On............Calories
MONDAY					Note........................
TUESDAY					
WEDNESDAY					
THURSDAY					
FRIDAY					
SATURDAY					
SUNDAY					

1 Week DASH Diet Base Control .... Calories					

Date	Breakfast	Lunch	Dinner	Snacks	DASH Diet Base On............Calories
MONDAY					Note........................
TUESDAY					
WEDNESDAY					
THURSDAY					
FRIDAY					
SATURDAY					
SUNDAY					

1 Week DASH Diet Base Control .... Calories					
Date	Breakfast	Lunch	Dinner	Snacks	DASH Diet Base On............Calories
MONDAY					Note..................... ....
TUESDAY					
WEDNESDAY					
THURSDAY					
FRIDAY					
SATURDAY					
SUNDAY					

1 Week DASH Diet Base Control .... Calories					
Date	Breakfast	Lunch	Dinner	Snacks	DASH Diet Base On...........Calories Note........................
MONDAY					
TUESDAY					
WEDNESDAY					
THURSDAY					
FRIDAY					
SATURDAY					
SUNDAY					

1 Week DASH Diet Base Control .... Calories					
Date	Breakfast	Lunch	Dinner	Snacks	DASH Diet Base On............Calories
MONDAY					Note......................
TUESDAY					
WEDNESDAY					
THURSDAY					
FRIDAY					
SATURDAY					
SUNDAY					

1 Week DASH Diet Base Control .... Calories

Date	Breakfast	Lunch	Dinner	Snacks	DASH Diet Base On.............Calories Note......................
MONDAY					
TUESDAY					
WEDNESDAY					
THURSDAY					
FRIDAY					
SATURDAY					
SUNDAY					

1 Week DASH Diet Base Control .... Calories

Date	Breakfast	Lunch	Dinner	Snacks	DASH Diet Base On.............Calories
					Note.......................
MONDAY					
TUESDAY					
WEDNESDAY					
THURSDAY					
FRIDAY					
SATURDAY					
SUNDAY					

1 Week DASH Diet Base Control					.... Calories
Date	Breakfast	Lunch	Dinner	Snacks	DASH Diet Base On............Calories
MONDAY					Note........................ ....
TUESDAY					
WEDNESDAY					
THURSDAY					
FRIDAY					
SATURDAY					
SUNDAY					

1 Week DASH Diet Base Control .... Calories				

Date	Breakfast	Lunch	Dinner	Snacks	DASH Diet Base On............Calories
MONDAY					Note........................ ....
TUESDAY					
WEDNESDAY					
THURSDAY					
FRIDAY					
SATURDAY					
SUNDAY					

1 Week DASH Diet Base Control .... Calories

Date	Breakfast	Lunch	Dinner	Snacks	DASH Diet
					Base On............Calories Note........................
MONDAY					
TUESDAY					
WEDNESDAY					
THURSDAY					
FRIDAY					
SATURDAY					
SUNDAY					

1 Week DASH Diet Base Control .... Calories					
Date	Breakfast	Lunch	Dinner	Snacks	DASH Diet Base On............Calories
MONDAY					Note........................
TUESDAY					
WEDNESDAY					
THURSDAY					
FRIDAY					
SATURDAY					
SUNDAY					

1 Week DASH Diet Base Control .... Calories

Date	Breakfast	Lunch	Dinner	Snacks	DASH Diet Base On............Calories
MONDAY					Note........................
TUESDAY					
WEDNESDAY					
THURSDAY					
FRIDAY					
SATURDAY					
SUNDAY					

1 Week DASH Diet Base Control .... Calories

Date	Breakfast	Lunch	Dinner	Snacks	DASH Diet Base On............Calories
MONDAY					Note................................
TUESDAY					
WEDNESDAY					
THURSDAY					
FRIDAY					
SATURDAY					
SUNDAY					

1 Week DASH Diet Base Control .... Calories					
Date	Breakfast	Lunch	Dinner	Snacks	DASH Diet Base On...........Calories
MONDAY					Note....................... ....
TUESDAY					
WEDNESDAY					
THURSDAY					
FRIDAY					
SATURDAY					
SUNDAY					

1 Week DASH Diet Base Control .... Calories

Date	Breakfast	Lunch	Dinner	Snacks	DASH Diet Base On.............Calories
MONDAY					Note.........................
TUESDAY					
WEDNESDAY					
THURSDAY					
FRIDAY					
SATURDAY					
SUNDAY					

1 Week DASH Diet Base Control............................... Calories

Date	Breakfast	Lunch	Dinner	Snacks	DASH Diet Base On............Calories
MONDAY					Note........................
TUESDAY					
WEDNESDAY					
THURSDAY					
FRIDAY					
SATURDAY					
SUNDAY					

1 Week DASH Diet Base Control .... Calories					
Date	Breakfast	Lunch	Dinner	Snacks	DASH Diet Base On............Calories Note........................
MONDAY					
TUESDAY					
WEDNESDAY					
THURSDAY					
FRIDAY					
SATURDAY					
SUNDAY					

1 Week DASH Diet Base Control .... Calories					
Date	Breakfast	Lunch	Dinner	Snacks	DASH Diet Base On............Calories
MONDAY					Note......................
TUESDAY					
WEDNESDAY					
THURSDAY					
FRIDAY					
SATURDAY					
SUNDAY					

1 Week DASH Diet Base Control					.... Calories
Date	Breakfast	Lunch	Dinner	Snacks	DASH Diet Base On............Calories
MONDAY					Note........................
TUESDAY					
WEDNESDAY					
THURSDAY					
FRIDAY					
SATURDAY					
SUNDAY					

1 Week DASH Diet Base Control .... Calories					
Date	Breakfast	Lunch	Dinner	Snacks	DASH Diet Base On............Calories Note.......................
MONDAY					
TUESDAY					
WEDNESDAY					
THURSDAY					
FRIDAY					
SATURDAY					
SUNDAY					

1 Week DASH Diet Base Control .... Calories

Date	Breakfast	Lunch	Dinner	Snacks	DASH Diet Base On............Calories
MONDAY					Note......................
TUESDAY					
WEDNESDAY					
THURSDAY					
FRIDAY					
SATURDAY					
SUNDAY					

1 Week DASH Diet Base Control .... Calories

Date	Breakfast	Lunch	Dinner	Snacks	DASH Diet Base On............Calories
MONDAY					Note........................
TUESDAY					
WEDNESDAY					
THURSDAY					
FRIDAY					
SATURDAY					
SUNDAY					

1 Week DASH Diet Base Control .... Calories					
Date	Breakfast	Lunch	Dinner	Snacks	DASH Diet Base On............Calories Note..........................
MONDAY					
TUESDAY					
WEDNESDAY					
THURSDAY					
FRIDAY					
SATURDAY					
SUNDAY					

1 Week DASH Diet Base Control .... Calories					
Date	Breakfast	Lunch	Dinner	Snacks	DASH Diet Base On............Calories
MONDAY					Note........................ ....
TUESDAY					
WEDNESDAY					
THURSDAY					
FRIDAY					
SATURDAY					
SUNDAY					

1 Week DASH Diet Base Control .... Calories					
Date	Breakfast	Lunch	Dinner	Snacks	DASH Diet Base On............Calories
MONDAY					Note........................
TUESDAY					
WEDNESDAY					
THURSDAY					
FRIDAY					
SATURDAY					
SUNDAY					

Date	Breakfast	Lunch	Dinner	Snacks	DASH Diet Base On............Calories
					Note....................... ....
MONDAY					
TUESDAY					
WEDNESDAY					
THURSDAY					
FRIDAY					
SATURDAY					
SUNDAY					

1 Week DASH Diet Base Control .... Calories

1 Week DASH Diet Base Control					.... Calories
Date	Breakfast	Lunch	Dinner	Snacks	DASH Diet Base On............Calories Note....................
MONDAY					
TUESDAY					
WEDNESDAY					
THURSDAY					
FRIDAY					
SATURDAY					
SUNDAY					

1 Week DASH Diet Base Control .... Calories

Date	Breakfast	Lunch	Dinner	Snacks	DASH Diet Base On............Calories
MONDAY					Note.......................
TUESDAY					
WEDNESDAY					
THURSDAY					
FRIDAY					
SATURDAY					
SUNDAY					

1 Week DASH Diet Base Control .... Calories					
Date	Breakfast	Lunch	Dinner	Snacks	DASH Diet Base On...........Calories
MONDAY					Note........................
TUESDAY					
WEDNESDAY					
THURSDAY					
FRIDAY					
SATURDAY					
SUNDAY					

1 Week DASH Diet Base Control .... Calories					
Date	Breakfast	Lunch	Dinner	Snacks	DASH Diet Base On............Calories
MONDAY					Note........................
TUESDAY					
WEDNESDAY					
THURSDAY					
FRIDAY					
SATURDAY					
SUNDAY					

1 Week DASH Diet Base Control .... Calories					
Date	Breakfast	Lunch	Dinner	Snacks	**DASH Diet** Base On............Calories
MONDAY					Note.......................
TUESDAY					
WEDNESDAY					
THURSDAY					
FRIDAY					
SATURDAY					
SUNDAY					

1 Week DASH Diet Base Control				.... Calories	

Date	Breakfast	Lunch	Dinner	Snacks	DASH Diet Base On............Calories
MONDAY					Note......................... ....
TUESDAY					
WEDNESDAY					
THURSDAY					
FRIDAY					
SATURDAY					
SUNDAY					

1 Week DASH Diet Base Control .... Calories					
Date	Breakfast	Lunch	Dinner	Snacks	DASH Diet Base On............Calories
MONDAY					Note......................... ....
TUESDAY					
WEDNESDAY					
THURSDAY					
FRIDAY					
SATURDAY					
SUNDAY					

1 Week DASH Diet Base Control .... Calories				

Date	Breakfast	Lunch	Dinner	Snacks	DASH Diet Base On............Calories
MONDAY					Note.........................
TUESDAY					
WEDNESDAY					
THURSDAY					
FRIDAY					
SATURDAY					
SUNDAY					

1 Week DASH Diet Base Control					.... Calories

Date	Breakfast	Lunch	Dinner	Snacks	DASH Diet
					Base On............Calories
MONDAY					Note........................
TUESDAY					
WEDNESDAY					
THURSDAY					
FRIDAY					
SATURDAY					
SUNDAY					

1 Week DASH Diet Base Control .... Calories

Date	Breakfast	Lunch	Dinner	Snacks	DASH Diet Base On............Calories
MONDAY					Note........................
TUESDAY					
WEDNESDAY					
THURSDAY					
FRIDAY					
SATURDAY					
SUNDAY					

1 Week DASH Diet Base Control .... Calories					
Date	Breakfast	Lunch	Dinner	Snacks	DASH Diet Base On............Calories Note......................
MONDAY					
TUESDAY					
WEDNESDAY					
THURSDAY					
FRIDAY					
SATURDAY					
SUNDAY					

1 Week DASH Diet Base Control .... Calories

Date	Breakfast	Lunch	Dinner	Snacks	DASH Diet Base On.............Calories
MONDAY					Note........................
TUESDAY					
WEDNESDAY					
THURSDAY					
FRIDAY					
SATURDAY					
SUNDAY					

<table>
<tr><td colspan="6">1 Week DASH Diet Base Control .... Calories</td></tr>
<tr><td>Date</td><td>Breakfast</td><td>Lunch</td><td>Dinner</td><td>Snacks</td><td>DASH Diet
Base On............Calories
Note......................</td></tr>
<tr><td>MONDAY</td><td></td><td></td><td></td><td></td><td></td></tr>
<tr><td>TUESDAY</td><td></td><td></td><td></td><td></td><td></td></tr>
<tr><td>WEDNESDAY</td><td></td><td></td><td></td><td></td><td></td></tr>
<tr><td>THURSDAY</td><td></td><td></td><td></td><td></td><td></td></tr>
<tr><td>FRIDAY</td><td></td><td></td><td></td><td></td><td></td></tr>
<tr><td>SATURDAY</td><td></td><td></td><td></td><td></td><td></td></tr>
<tr><td>SUNDAY</td><td></td><td></td><td></td><td></td><td></td></tr>
</table>

1 Week DASH Diet Base Control .... Calories

Date	Breakfast	Lunch	Dinner	Snacks	DASH Diet Base On............Calories
MONDAY					Note........................
TUESDAY					
WEDNESDAY					
THURSDAY					
FRIDAY					
SATURDAY					
SUNDAY					

1 Week DASH Diet Base Control					.... Calories
Date	Breakfast	Lunch	Dinner	Snacks	DASH Diet Base On.............Calories
MONDAY					Note......................... ....
TUESDAY					
WEDNESDAY					
THURSDAY					
FRIDAY					
SATURDAY					
SUNDAY					

1 Week DASH Diet Base Control .... Calories					
Date	Breakfast	Lunch	Dinner	Snacks	DASH Diet Base On............Calories
MONDAY					Note........................
TUESDAY					
WEDNESDAY					
THURSDAY					
FRIDAY					
SATURDAY					
SUNDAY					

1 Week DASH Diet Base Control .... Calories					

Date	Breakfast	Lunch	Dinner	Snacks	DASH Diet Base On..............Calories
MONDAY					Note......................... ....
TUESDAY					
WEDNESDAY					
THURSDAY					
FRIDAY					
SATURDAY					
SUNDAY					

1 Week DASH Diet Base Control .... Calories					
Date	Breakfast	Lunch	Dinner	Snacks	DASH Diet Base On............Calories Note........................
MONDAY					
TUESDAY					
WEDNESDAY					
THURSDAY					
FRIDAY					
SATURDAY					
SUNDAY					

1 Week DASH Diet Base Control .... Calories					

Date	Breakfast	Lunch	Dinner	Snacks	DASH Diet Base On............Calories
MONDAY					Note.......................
TUESDAY					
WEDNESDAY					
THURSDAY					
FRIDAY					
SATURDAY					
SUNDAY					

1 Week DASH Diet Base Control					.... Calories
Date	Breakfast	Lunch	Dinner	Snacks	DASH Diet Base On............Calories
MONDAY					Note.........................
TUESDAY					
WEDNESDAY					
THURSDAY					
FRIDAY					
SATURDAY					
SUNDAY					

1 Week DASH Diet Base Control .... Calories					
Date	Breakfast	Lunch	Dinner	Snacks	DASH Diet Base On............Calories
MONDAY					Note........................
TUESDAY					
WEDNESDAY					
THURSDAY					
FRIDAY					
SATURDAY					
SUNDAY					

1 Week DASH Diet Base Control				.... Calories	
Date	Breakfast	Lunch	Dinner	Snacks	DASH Diet Base On...........Calories
MONDAY					Note.........................
TUESDAY					
WEDNESDAY					
THURSDAY					
FRIDAY					
SATURDAY					
SUNDAY					

1 Week DASH Diet Base Control .... Calories				

Date	Breakfast	Lunch	Dinner	Snacks	DASH Diet Base On............Calories
MONDAY					Note......................
TUESDAY					
WEDNESDAY					
THURSDAY					
FRIDAY					
SATURDAY					
SUNDAY					

1 Week DASH Diet Base Control .... Calories					
Date	Breakfast	Lunch	Dinner	Snacks	DASH Diet Base On.............Calories
MONDAY					Note........................ ....
TUESDAY					
WEDNESDAY					
THURSDAY					
FRIDAY					
SATURDAY					
SUNDAY					

1 Week DASH Diet Base Control					.... Calories
Date	Breakfast	Lunch	Dinner	Snacks	**DASH Diet** Base On.............Calories
MONDAY					Note........................ ....
TUESDAY					
WEDNESDAY					
THURSDAY					
FRIDAY					
SATURDAY					
SUNDAY					

1 Week DASH Diet Base Control .... Calories					
Date	Breakfast	Lunch	Dinner	Snacks	DASH Diet Base On............Calories
MONDAY					Note......................... ....
TUESDAY					
WEDNESDAY					
THURSDAY					
FRIDAY					
SATURDAY					
SUNDAY					

1 Week DASH Diet Base Control .... Calories					

Date	Breakfast	Lunch	Dinner	Snacks	DASH Diet Base On.............Calories
MONDAY					Note........................ ....
TUESDAY					
WEDNESDAY					
THURSDAY					
FRIDAY					
SATURDAY					
SUNDAY					

1 Week DASH Diet Base Control				.... Calories	
Date	Breakfast	Lunch	Dinner	Snacks	DASH Diet Base On............Calories
MONDAY					Note...................... ....
TUESDAY					
WEDNESDAY					
THURSDAY					
FRIDAY					
SATURDAY					
SUNDAY					

Date	Breakfast	Lunch	Dinner	Snacks	DASH Diet Base On............Calories
MONDAY					Note.....................
TUESDAY					
WEDNESDAY					
THURSDAY					
FRIDAY					
SATURDAY					
SUNDAY					

1 Week DASH Diet Base Control .... **Calories**

1 Week DASH Diet Base Control .... Calories					
Date	Breakfast	Lunch	Dinner	Snacks	DASH Diet Base On............Calories
MONDAY					Note......................
TUESDAY					
WEDNESDAY					
THURSDAY					
FRIDAY					
SATURDAY					
SUNDAY					

1 Week DASH Diet Base Control .... Calories				
Date	Breakfast	Lunch	Dinner	Snacks	DASH Diet Base On...........Calories
MONDAY					Note..................... ....
TUESDAY					
WEDNESDAY					
THURSDAY					
FRIDAY					
SATURDAY					
SUNDAY					

1 Week DASH Diet Base Control					.... Calories
Date	Breakfast	Lunch	Dinner	Snacks	DASH Diet Base On.............Calories
MONDAY					Note........................
TUESDAY					
WEDNESDAY					
THURSDAY					
FRIDAY					
SATURDAY					
SUNDAY					

1 Week DASH Diet Base Control .... Calories				

Date	Breakfast	Lunch	Dinner	Snacks	DASH Diet Base On............Calories
MONDAY					Note........................ ....
TUESDAY					
WEDNESDAY					
THURSDAY					
FRIDAY					
SATURDAY					
SUNDAY					

1 Week DASH Diet Base Control .... Calories

Date	Breakfast	Lunch	Dinner	Snacks	DASH Diet Base On............Calories
MONDAY					Note........................
TUESDAY					
WEDNESDAY					
THURSDAY					
FRIDAY					
SATURDAY					
SUNDAY					

1 Week DASH Diet Base Control .... Calories					
Date	Breakfast	Lunch	Dinner	Snacks	DASH Diet Base On.............Calories Note.........................
MONDAY					
TUESDAY					
WEDNESDAY					
THURSDAY					
FRIDAY					
SATURDAY					
SUNDAY					

1 Week DASH Diet Base Control				.... Calories	
Date	Breakfast	Lunch	Dinner	Snacks	DASH Diet Base On............Calories
MONDAY					Note.........................
TUESDAY					
WEDNESDAY					
THURSDAY					
FRIDAY					
SATURDAY					
SUNDAY					

1 Week DASH Diet Base Control .... Calories

Date	Breakfast	Lunch	Dinner	Snacks	DASH Diet
					Base On............Calories
MONDAY					Note.........................
TUESDAY					
WEDNESDAY					
THURSDAY					
FRIDAY					
SATURDAY					
SUNDAY					

1 Week DASH Diet Base Control .... Calories

Date	Breakfast	Lunch	Dinner	Snacks	DASH Diet Base On............Calories
MONDAY					Note.........................
TUESDAY					
WEDNESDAY					
THURSDAY					
FRIDAY					
SATURDAY					
SUNDAY					

1 Week DASH Diet Base Control .... Calories					
Date	Breakfast	Lunch	Dinner	Snacks	DASH Diet Base On............Calories
MONDAY					Note.........................
TUESDAY					
WEDNESDAY					
THURSDAY					
FRIDAY					
SATURDAY					
SUNDAY					

1 Week DASH Diet Base Control .... Calories					
Date	Breakfast	Lunch	Dinner	Snacks	DASH Diet Base On.............Calories
MONDAY					Note....................... ....
TUESDAY					
WEDNESDAY					
THURSDAY					
FRIDAY					
SATURDAY					
SUNDAY					

1 Week DASH Diet Base Control .... Calories

Date	Breakfast	Lunch	Dinner	Snacks	DASH Diet Base On............Calories
MONDAY					Note...................... ....
TUESDAY					
WEDNESDAY					
THURSDAY					
FRIDAY					
SATURDAY					
SUNDAY					

1 Week DASH Diet Base Control .... Calories

Date	Breakfast	Lunch	Dinner	Snacks	DASH Diet Base On............Calories
MONDAY					Note.......................
TUESDAY					
WEDNESDAY					
THURSDAY					
FRIDAY					
SATURDAY					
SUNDAY					

<table>
<tr><td colspan="6">1 Week DASH Diet Base Control .... Calories</td></tr>
<tr><td>Date</td><td>Breakfast</td><td>Lunch</td><td>Dinner</td><td>Snacks</td><td>DASH Diet
Base On............Calories</td></tr>
<tr><td>MONDAY</td><td></td><td></td><td></td><td></td><td>Note........................
........................</td></tr>
<tr><td>TUESDAY</td><td></td><td></td><td></td><td></td><td></td></tr>
<tr><td>WEDNESDAY</td><td></td><td></td><td></td><td></td><td></td></tr>
<tr><td>THURSDAY</td><td></td><td></td><td></td><td></td><td></td></tr>
<tr><td>FRIDAY</td><td></td><td></td><td></td><td></td><td></td></tr>
<tr><td>SATURDAY</td><td></td><td></td><td></td><td></td><td></td></tr>
<tr><td>SUNDAY</td><td></td><td></td><td></td><td></td><td></td></tr>
</table>

1 Week DASH Diet Base Control .... Calories					
Date	Breakfast	Lunch	Dinner	Snacks	DASH Diet Base On............Calories Note........................
MONDAY					
TUESDAY					
WEDNESDAY					
THURSDAY					
FRIDAY					
SATURDAY					
SUNDAY					

1 Week DASH Diet Base Control					.... Calories
Date	Breakfast	Lunch	Dinner	Snacks	DASH Diet Base On.............Calories
MONDAY					Note.......................
TUESDAY					
WEDNESDAY					
THURSDAY					
FRIDAY					
SATURDAY					
SUNDAY					

1 Week DASH Diet Base Control				.... Calories	
Date	Breakfast	Lunch	Dinner	Snacks	DASH Diet Base On............Calories
MONDAY					Note......................... ....
TUESDAY					
WEDNESDAY					
THURSDAY					
FRIDAY					
SATURDAY					
SUNDAY					

1 Week DASH Diet Base Control .... Calories					
Date	Breakfast	Lunch	Dinner	Snacks	DASH Diet Base On............Calories
MONDAY					Note.................. ....
TUESDAY					
WEDNESDAY					
THURSDAY					
FRIDAY					
SATURDAY					
SUNDAY					

1 Week DASH Diet Base Control .... Calories					
Date	Breakfast	Lunch	Dinner	Snacks	DASH Diet Base On.............Calories Note........................
MONDAY					
TUESDAY					
WEDNESDAY					
THURSDAY					
FRIDAY					
SATURDAY					
SUNDAY					

1 Week DASH Diet Base Control .... Calories					
Date	Breakfast	Lunch	Dinner	Snacks	DASH Diet Base On............Calories
MONDAY					Note......................
TUESDAY					
WEDNESDAY					
THURSDAY					
FRIDAY					
SATURDAY					
SUNDAY					

1 Week DASH Diet Base Control				.... Calories	

Date	Breakfast	Lunch	Dinner	Snacks	DASH Diet Base On.............Calories
MONDAY					Note........................
TUESDAY					
WEDNESDAY					
THURSDAY					
FRIDAY					
SATURDAY					
SUNDAY					

1 Week DASH Diet Base Control .... Calories					
Date	Breakfast	Lunch	Dinner	Snacks	DASH Diet Base On............Calories
MONDAY					Note......................... ....
TUESDAY					
WEDNESDAY					
THURSDAY					
FRIDAY					
SATURDAY					
SUNDAY					

1 Week DASH Diet Base Control.. Calories					

Date	Breakfast	Lunch	Dinner	Snacks	DASH Diet Base On............Calories
MONDAY					Note........................
TUESDAY					
WEDNESDAY					
THURSDAY					
FRIDAY					
SATURDAY					
SUNDAY					

| 1 Week DASH Diet Base Control | | | | | .... Calories |
Date	Breakfast	Lunch	Dinner	Snacks	DASH Diet Base On.............Calories
MONDAY					Note.........................
TUESDAY					
WEDNESDAY					
THURSDAY					
FRIDAY					
SATURDAY					
SUNDAY					

1 Week DASH Diet Base Control				.... Calories	
Date	Breakfast	Lunch	Dinner	Snacks	DASH Diet Base On............Calories
MONDAY					Note........................ ....
TUESDAY					
WEDNESDAY					
THURSDAY					
FRIDAY					
SATURDAY					
SUNDAY					

1 Week DASH Diet Base Control .... Calories					
Date	Breakfast	Lunch	Dinner	Snacks	DASH Diet Base On............Calories
MONDAY					Note........................
TUESDAY					
WEDNESDAY					
THURSDAY					
FRIDAY					
SATURDAY					
SUNDAY					

1 Week DASH Diet Base Control .... Calories

Date	Breakfast	Lunch	Dinner	Snacks	DASH Diet Base On.............Calories
MONDAY					Note.........................
TUESDAY					
WEDNESDAY					
THURSDAY					
FRIDAY					
SATURDAY					
SUNDAY					

1 Week DASH Diet Base Control .... Calories

Date	Breakfast	Lunch	Dinner	Snacks	DASH Diet Base On.............Calories
MONDAY					Note........................ ....
TUESDAY					
WEDNESDAY					
THURSDAY					
FRIDAY					
SATURDAY					
SUNDAY					

1 Week DASH Diet Base Control .... Calories

Date	Breakfast	Lunch	Dinner	Snacks	DASH Diet Base On............Calories
MONDAY					Note........................
TUESDAY					
WEDNESDAY					
THURSDAY					
FRIDAY					
SATURDAY					
SUNDAY					

1 Week DASH Diet Base Control					.... Calories
Date	Breakfast	Lunch	Dinner	Snacks	DASH Diet Base On............Calories
MONDAY					Note.....................
TUESDAY					
WEDNESDAY					
THURSDAY					
FRIDAY					
SATURDAY					
SUNDAY					

<table>
<tr><td colspan="6">1 Week DASH Diet Base Control .... Calories</td></tr>
<tr><td>Date</td><td>Breakfast</td><td>Lunch</td><td>Dinner</td><td>Snacks</td><td>DASH Diet
Base On............Calories</td></tr>
<tr><td>MONDAY</td><td></td><td></td><td></td><td></td><td>Note.......................</td></tr>
<tr><td>TUESDAY</td><td></td><td></td><td></td><td></td><td></td></tr>
<tr><td>WEDNESDAY</td><td></td><td></td><td></td><td></td><td></td></tr>
<tr><td>THURSDAY</td><td></td><td></td><td></td><td></td><td></td></tr>
<tr><td>FRIDAY</td><td></td><td></td><td></td><td></td><td></td></tr>
<tr><td>SATURDAY</td><td></td><td></td><td></td><td></td><td></td></tr>
<tr><td>SUNDAY</td><td></td><td></td><td></td><td></td><td></td></tr>
</table>

1 Week DASH Diet Base Control .... Calories					
Date	Breakfast	Lunch	Dinner	Snacks	DASH Diet Base On............Calories Note........................
MONDAY					
TUESDAY					
WEDNESDAY					
THURSDAY					
FRIDAY					
SATURDAY					
SUNDAY